SORE THROAT

Methods for Relieving Throat Pain and Maintaining Good Health

CHAD BRUNO

Table of Contents

Introductory

Pain, discomfort, or irritation in the throat, especially during swallowing, characterizes a common medical ailment known as a sore throat. Environmental factors (such as exposure to smoking or pollutants), allergies, or other irritants can all play a role, as can virus infections (like the common cold or flu) or bacterial infections (like strep throat). A sore throat can cause mild to severe pain and discomfort, as well as additional symptoms including scratchiness, dryness, and hoarseness.

When infections are to blame for a person's sore throat, additional symptoms may also present themselves. How you treat a sore throat depends on what's causing it. In most cases, a sore throat caused by a virus will go away with rest and over-the-counter medications, whereas a sore throat caused by bacteria may require antibiotics. Pain medicines, throat lozenges, and calming beverages like hot tea with honey are all commonly used to manage symptoms. A doctor should be consulted if a sore throat lasts more than a few days or is accompanied by other severe symptoms.

CHAPTER ONE
A Guide to Throat Pain

The causes, symptoms, diagnosis, and treatment choices for sore throats must all be known in order to effectively deal with this frequent medical issue. Here is a more in-depth summary:

1. **Viral Infections:** The common cold, influenza, and the Epstein-Barr virus (responsible for infectious mononucleosis) are the most prevalent causes of sore throats.

Strep throat, caused by the bacterium Streptococcus, is an example of a bacterial infection.

Sore throats can also be caused by other types of germs.

Sore throats can be brought on by being subjected to environmental irritants like tobacco smoke, pollution, or dry air.

An itchy throat may be the result of an allergic reaction to pollen, pet dander, or another allergen.

Acid from the stomach can leak up into the esophagus and cause a persistent painful throat in people with gastroesophageal reflux disease (GERD).

Excessive shouting, talking, or singing can cause strain on the vocal cords and result in a sore throat.

2. Throat pain or discomfort, especially during swallowing.

• Throat irritation, dryness, or scratchiness.

• A hoarse or raspy voice.

• Neck lymph nodes that are swollen.

Itchy coughing.

• Congestion and sneezing.

• Nose bleed.

An infection-related fever.

3. Diagnosis:

A sore throats cause can be determined by a doctor after a thorough physical examination and, in some situations, a throat sample sent to the lab for testing.

• Your symptoms, their severity, and how long they've lasted may all factor into the diagnosis.

4. Viral sore throats are usually treated with bed rest, plenty of fluids, and nonprescription pain medications. Gargling with warm saltwater, using throat lozenges, and drinking soothing beverages like hot tea with honey can all help.

• Sore Throats Caused by Bacteria: Antibiotics are used to treat strep throat, a bacterial illness.

In any case, home remedies like increasing fluid intake, utilizing a humidifier, and avoiding irritants like smoking will help alleviate symptoms. You can also try taking some over-the-counter painkillers.

Sore throats can be avoided by taking preventative measures, such as regularly washing your hands and staying away from people who are sick.

If you have a severe sore throat that lasts longer than a few days or if it is followed by other worrying symptoms like trouble breathing, extreme pain, or high fever, you should seek medical attention. If you visit a doctor, they can assist you figure out what's wrong and how to treat it.

Symptoms and Indicators

Changes or indicators of a medical condition, illness, or disease that are both objective and perceptual are known as signs and symptoms. They provide crucial information for doctors to use in making diagnoses and formulating treatment plans. Some typical symptoms include:

1. A rise in core body temperature, or fever, is a common symptom of infection or inflammation.

2. Pain is characterized by localized discomfort or suffering and can have several origins including tissue damage, inflammation, or illness.

3. Fatigue is a sign of many different diseases and disorders, such as infections, chronic illnesses, and mental health problems.

4. Headache: Pain or discomfort in the head might be related to tension, sinus problems, migraines, or other causes.

5. Nausea and vomiting can arise from many different health problems, including those in the digestive system, food poisoning, pregnancy, and others.

6. A cough is a symptom of many respiratory illnesses, including the common cold, influenza, and even bronchitis and pneumonia.

7. Conditions affecting the respiratory system, the heart, or other health concerns can all contribute to shortness of breath.

8. Edema (Swelling) is caused by fluid retention and can be a symptom of a number of different medical issues, including those affecting the heart, kidneys, and liver.

9. Allergic reactions, infections, autoimmune illnesses, and irritants are all potential causes of a skin rash.

10. Arthritis, autoimmune illnesses, and injuries are only some of the causes of joint pain, stiffness, and edema.

11. A painful throat may be the result of a viral or bacterial illness, an allergic reaction, or exposure to an allergen.

12. Chest discomfort: Chest discomfort can be a sign of heart difficulties, lung issues, gastrointestinal diseases, or even anxiety.

13. Diarrhea, constipation, bloody stools, or other alterations in bowel habits may be symptomatic of underlying digestive or other health problems.

14. Urinary Tract Infections, Kidney Disease, and Other Conditions Can Be Identified by Alterations in Urine Flow, Urinary Pain, and Urine Color and Odor.

15. Depression, anxiety, irritability, and other mood-related symptoms may indicate a neurological or mental health issue.

16. Conditions including Alzheimer's disease, dementia, and stress have been related to memory, cognitive, and focus difficulties.

17. Unexpected shifts in body weight might indicate a number of serious health issues.

18. Visual Changes: Blurred vision, double vision, or changes in visual acuity can signal eye diseases, diabetes, or neurological difficulties.

19. Hearing Loss: Ear infections, aging, and other ear-related disorders can cause either gradual or sudden hearing loss.

Keep in mind that many symptoms are generic and may indicate a variety of health issues. A medical practitioner should evaluate and diagnose any symptoms that continue or worsen over time.

CHAPTER TWO
Natural Cures

Common health problems and associated discomfort can often be alleviated with the use of simple, all-natural home remedies. In most cases, they shouldn't be used in place of getting checked out by a doctor, but they can help with mild problems in the short term. Home treatments for a few prevalent ailments are as follows:

1. Throat Ache:

Use a saltwater gargle with warm water.

• Drink warm herbal teas with honey.

You may get throat lozenges and sprays from the drugstore.

2. Cough:

• Sip on some hot liquids, like broth or herbal tea.

• Honey and lemon are a traditional remedy for coughs. Try a cup of hot tea or water.

Humidifiers can be used to increase humidity levels in a room.

3. Congestion:

• Inhale vapor from a basin of hot water with a cloth over your head.

Clearing nasal passages with a saline nasal spray or saline nasal rinse is a viable option.

4. Headache:

• Place an ice pack on your head or neck to help you relax.

Relax in a calm, dark place.

Keep drinking water.

5. Nausea:

• If you're feeling queasy, try some ginger tea or chews.

Be sure to drink enough of water or other non-cloudy fluids to prevent dehydration.

• Eat bland, easily digestible items like crackers or toast.

6. Sunburn:

Use aloe vera gel on the wound.

• Apply cold baths or compresses to your skin.

• Drink plenty of water to speed up recovery.

7. Feeling Queasy:

Clear liquids such as ginger ale or broth should be consumed.

Tea made from either peppermint or ginger helps calm an upset stomach.

Don't eat anything too heavy, greasy, or spicy.

8. Slight Burns:

• Apply cool running water to the burn for a few minutes to alleviate the pain.

• Use a burn ointment or aloe vera gel that you can get at a drugstore.

• Wrap it in a clean, adhesive-free bandage.

9. Acne:

Use a mild, non-comedogenic cleanser to wash your face.

Use a mask made of honey and cinnamon.

Spot-treat with tea tree oil.

10. Injuries of a Minimal Nature:

Use a gentle soap and water to wash the wound.

• Apply an over-the-counter antibiotic ointment.

Put a clean bandage over it.

11. Neck Pain:

Warm the neck area with a heating pad or compress.

Possible aid from light neck exercises and stretches.

12. Insomnia:

Develop a soothing nighttime ritual.

Don't use devices or drink caffeine near bedtime.

Teas made from herbs, including chamomile, are known to provide calming effects.

13. Poor Hygiene:

Don't let plaque buildup on your tongue and teeth.

• Rinse your mouth out with mouthwash or a solution of baking soda and water.

Keep drinking water to avoid having a dry mouth.

14. Hiccups:

• Don't breathe for a couple of minutes.

• Take a few sips from a glass of ice water.

• Gargle with cold water.

Keep in mind that most home remedies are only appropriate for treating temporary and mild problems. If you have a serious or ongoing health issue, you should see a doctor to get a correct diagnosis and treatment plan. Be wary of trying new treatments if you have allergies or sensitivities; if you have any negative responses, stop taking the product immediately.

Health Care Procedures

Medical treatments are actions administered by medical practitioners for the purpose of identifying, treating, and preventing illness. Medication, surgery, therapeutic interventions, and even changes in way of life can all be part of the treatment spectrum. The specific course of medical treatment for a given ailment is contingent upon the nature and severity of that condition.

1. Medications:

Drugs available only with a doctor's prescription can be used to treat infections, control the symptoms of chronic diseases, and solve other health problems. Antibiotics, analgesics, blood pressure medications, and anticoagulants are just a few examples.

OTC drugs are available without a doctor's prescription and are useful for treating common ailments like the common cold, allergies, and moderate pain.

2. Operative Techniques:

• Surgical intervention could be required to get rid of malignancies, fix broken organs or tissues, or fix structural faults. Among the most often performed operations are appendectomy, joint replacement, and heart bypass.

3. Rehab and physical therapy:

Exercises, stretches, and manual therapies are some of the tools used by physical therapists to aid patients in their recovery from accidents, surgeries, or ongoing medical issues.

4.Treatment with Radiation:

High-energy rays are used by radiation oncologists to specifically target and kill cancer cells. It's a standard part of cancer care.

5. Chemotherapy:

Chemotherapy refers to the employment of medications to either directly kill cancer cells or inhibit their growth. It's typically given in cycles.

6. Immunotherapy:

By strengthening the immune system, immunotherapy can be

used to combat serious illnesses like cancer.

7. Dialysis:

Dialysis is a procedure used to remove waste products and excess fluids from the blood of people who have renal failure or decreased kidney function.

8. Donating an Organ:

Kidney, liver, heart, and lung transplants are all possible treatments for patients with end-stage organ failure.

9. Therapies for Mental Illness:

Treatments for mental health issues may include psychotherapy (talk therapy), medication, and lifestyle modifications to control symptoms.

10. Vaccinations:

Vaccines are preventative measures that aid in the development of immunity to disease. The flu, measles, and a virus called COVID-19 can all be avoided with their help.

11. To intervene physically:

These include methods like acupuncture, chiropractic care, and massage therapy, which may be used to manage pain and certain health concerns.

12. Adjustments to Your Way of Life:

Doctors and other medical professionals regularly stress the importance of adopting healthier habits for patients. Changes in diet, physical activity, nicotine replacement therapy, and stress management are all possibilities.

13. Physical and Occupational Therapy for Recuperation

Recovery and regaining mobility and function following illness, surgery, or injury are aided by these therapies.

14. Remedy for Breathing:

Respiratory therapists help people who have trouble breathing by giving them treatments like breathing exercises and oxygen therapy.

15. HRT is used to treat hormonal imbalances caused by menopause or other hormone-related diseases or disorders.

If you're not sure what kind of medical attention might be best for your condition, go to a doctor. When making treatment recommendations, medical professionals think on the patient's medical history, the severity of the ailment, any possible side effects, and the patient's preferences. The field of medicine is ever-evolving, with new methods and therapies being discovered to enhance health and well-being for patients.

CHAPTER THREE
Avoiding a Coughing Fit

A sore throat can be avoided by practicing excellent hygiene and avoiding activities that increase the likelihood of developing an infection or irritation of the throat. To avoid getting a sore throat, use these measures:

1. Regular hand washing with soap and water can help prevent the spread of germs and disease. One of the best methods to stop the transmission of illness is to practice good hand hygiene.

2. Don't go too close to sick people, especially if they have a respiratory

illness like a cold or the flu. Infectious agents such as viruses and bacteria can transmit from person to person.

3. If you want to stop the spread of germs from your cough or sneeze, use a tissue or your elbow to cover your mouth and nose. Please flush tissues and wash your hands after use.

4. To avoid getting a sore throat, practice good oral hygiene by brushing and flossing daily. It's possible that sore throats are caused by bacteria in the mouth.

5. Hydrate well to prevent dryness and irritation of the throat. If you frequently experience sore throats as a result of dry air in your home, you may want to invest in a humidifier.

6. Limit Your Exposure to Potential Irritants: Smoke, Pollutants, Etc. Inflammation of the throat is a common side effect of smoking and secondhand smoke.

7. Consult an allergist to determine and treat the causes of your postnasal drip if you suffer from allergies. A painful throat is a common symptom of an allergic reaction.

8. Vaccinations: Protect yourself from potentially dangerous diseases by getting the flu shot and the meningococcal vaccine. Infections that cause sore throats are infrequently contracted thanks to vaccinations.

9. Eat Well A diet rich in fruits and vegetables can help strengthen your immune system and enhance your overall health, so be sure to include lots of these foods in your daily meals.

10. Stay Active: Regular physical activity can assist preserve excellent health and a robust immune system.

11. Reduce your stress levels; being overly anxious can lower your resistance to illness. Try some relaxation techniques like yoga, deep breathing, or meditation to calm yourself down.

12. Indoor air quality can be maintained and pollutants reduced with proper ventilation in the house or office.

13. Don't share your food, drink, or other personal goods with other people, especially if they appear to be ill.

14. Keep abreast of current health advice and precautions, especially during flu and other disease epidemics. To lessen the possibility of infection, stick to the rules.

15. Sore throats can be caused by sexually transmitted diseases (STIs), thus it's important to take precautions when engaging in sexual activity.

16. Be aware of local health advisories and take measures to protect yourself from infectious diseases before you visit.

Preventing sore throats often includes maintaining excellent general health and minimizing exposure to possible irritants and infectious agents. If your sore throat is chronic or severe, or if you have a medical condition that predisposes you to throat problems, you should seek the advice of a medical practitioner.

People of all ages and walks of life are susceptible to developing a sore throat, but certain populations may have additional elements to consider. Here are some group-specific things to keep in mind when dealing with sore throats:

1. Youngsters and Newborns:

• Children are more likely to contract viral infections that can cause sore throats, especially those who spend time in child care or school environments.

• Antibiotics may be necessary to treat strep throat, which is prevalent in children.

• Because kids can't always explain how they feel, it's up to adults to keep an eye out for things like a high temperature, a reluctance to eat or drink, and other discomforts.

• Medications with a pediatric formulation should be utilized, and dosage correctly is essential.

2. Expectant Mothers:

• Pregnant women should exercise caution when using any kind of medication, whether it be over-the-counter or prescribed, and should always check with their doctor first.

• Some infections pose hazards to both the mother and the growing fetus if not treated promptly, thus prenatal care is a must.

3. Senior Citizens:

• The elderly may have poorer immune systems, leaving them more susceptible to infections, including those causing sore throats.

• Chronic sore throats can be caused by age-related disorders such gastroesophageal reflux disease (GERD).

Healthcare practitioners should take into account the increased likelihood of medication interactions and side effects in the elderly.

4. Those having a compromised immune system:

• People with weakened immune systems due to HIV/AIDS, cancer treatment, or organ transplantation are at increased risk for developing severe and persistent infections.

• Infections in this population can be life-threatening, thus early diagnosis and effective treatment are critical.

5. Persons with Allergies:

Postnasal drip from allergens like pollen, pet dander, or dust mites can irritate the throat and lead to a painful throat in people who are allergic to these substances.

Sore throats can be avoided to some degree with the help of allergy management tactics and drugs.

6. The Healthcare Team:

• Healthcare workers are more likely to catch infections that cause sore throats because of their frequent contact with ill patients.

• Hand cleanliness and the use of protective gear are just two of several infection control procedures that should be strictly adhered to in order to reduce the potential for harm.

7. Athletes:

• Close contact between teammates might increase the risk of strep throat and other diseases among athletes, especially in contact sports.

You can lessen your exposure by doing things like not sharing water bottles or other items.

8. People who are dealing with Long-Term Illness:

Recurrent sore throats may be a symptom of a more serious problem in those with chronic diseases such as gastroesophageal reflux disease (GERD) or autoimmune disorders.

Sore throats can be avoided by taking care of the underlying cause and avoiding any precipitating factors.

It is crucial to recognize specific risk factors, anticipate probable consequences, and seek timely medical intervention in vulnerable populations. Medical professionals should modify their methods and treatments to better serve these populations. In addition, immunizations and other preventative measures like proper cleanliness are essential to lowering the rate of sore throats among vulnerable groups.

Conclusion

Throat pain has many potential origins, including viral and bacterial infections, the environment, allergies, and more. Sore throats can be difficult to deal with and prevent if you don't know what causes them and what the warning signals are.

Minor health problems, such as a sore throat, can often be alleviated with home remedies. Good dental hygiene, minimizing irritants, and reducing dryness in the air are all part of these measures. However, it is essential to seek competent medical advice and treatment for persistent or severe sore throats.

A sore throat can be treated medically in a number of ways, from medication and surgery to therapy and lifestyle changes. The severity and origin of the ailment are primary considerations in selecting a course of treatment.

Sore throats can be avoided with regular hygiene, up-to-date vaccinations, and a nutritious diet and exercise routine. Children, pregnant women, the elderly, and people with compromised immune systems may have different needs and concerns than the general population when it comes to sore throats. Prevention and treatment strategies must be individualized to address these differences.

In all situations, early diagnosis and adequate care play a crucial role in lowering the discomfort and health concerns associated with sore throats. The negative effects of sore throats can be lessened if people observe healthy habits and get medical help when it's needed.

THE END